VEGETARIANISM
UNMASKED

VEGETARIANISM UNMASKED

Unmasking the Truth About Vegetarianism

Buddy Poy

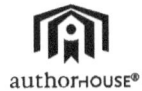

authorHOUSE®

AuthorHouse™
1663 Liberty Drive
Bloomington, IN 47403
www.authorhouse.com
Phone: 1-800-839-8640

First published by AuthorHouse   05/14/2011

ISBN: 978-1-4634-0877-0 (sc)
ISBN: 978-1-4634-0876-3 (dj)
ISBN: 978-1-4634-0875-6 (ebk)

Library of Congress Control Number: 2011908028

Printed in the United States of America

Table of Contents

Introduction

Vegetarianism today is a very hot topic and filled with lots of emotions among people of all level of society all over the world, there are vegetarian societies in all major countries and cities around the globe. Vegetarians today really believe that the best and only diet is the vegetarian diet for all of humanity, that it is the best diet for humans, animals, and the eco-system. Basing their opinion by saying among many things that man is a vegetarian animal by nature, and stating that man physiologically is a vegetarian animal. This view point will be fully addressed in full in later chapters. Others believe that man is an omnivores animal by nature and they base their conclusion in new information from medicine, science, and physiological findings. All this talk about being a vegetarian because the vegetarian diet is the best diet for man is not the main reason among vegetarians themselves for being a vegetarian. The main reason I believe is the humane reason for not consuming animals and their by—products saying that its wrong and unnecessary for man to kill animals for their own personal needs, and by this action causing extreme damage to the animal kingdom, the vegetable kingdom, and the environment through the mass production of animals in today's farming systems. This idea has many issues that we will discuss throughout the book and with it many many surprises. I believe that more than 75% of vegetarians are vegetarians because of this reason, and not the dietary reason with all its difficulties for the western man, and stating that we should live life without doing harm to the animal kingdom a process that we will see how difficult and almost impossible it is to carry out once we understand what exactly is the animal kingdom. It should be realized that there must be a line of demarcation into how far we can go in order to comply with this task without causing the harm that usually comes with such a difficult decision. That is why I am going to explain the vastness of what is the animal kingdom. Together we will try to understand the reality and complexity of such an important topic that's causing so much commotion among people today. This book will not only deal with vegetarianism on a dietary level but mainly on the effect that it has on the individual on an emotional, physiological, and especially social level where the real difficulty exists. I would like for everybody to know that I am not only talking about this topic based on research but from my own experience as a vegetarian for almost three decades.

I will also deal with what I think is one of the most important issue when it comes to vegetarianism nutrients and vitamins. I will go into a complete detail of their importance and function in relation to the physical body and its need.

Let us ask is vegetarianism only a diet of many levels or is it a way of life for the individuals that adapt to its principals. We know that this is something that affects the total nature and the way of living for the individual that is a vegetarian, especially to the western man who is totally dependent to animal flesh and its by-product. The question whether to be a vegetarian or to eat meat is one that is in the minds of many people today. Some are still consumers of meat and users of their by—products, while others are vegans that seem to believe that the meat eaters are evil and can't grow spiritually or make any advancement in any religious path, and that they are totally selfish when it comes to nature, animals, humanity, and the ecological situation of the world today. This is a topic that has involved the opinion of many occult schools, religions, spiritual path, Initiates, philosophers, famous people, scientist, and people of regular walk of life. The opinion among them has been divided some in favor of meat eating or mixed diet and others on the vegetarian diet remember this is a topic that has been around for thousands of years especially in the east. There must be many ways to approach this topic with all its intricate complexity and vast opinions among people today. I really want for everybody to understand that I am not a scholar writing a text book, but one who is writing about a very important topic that is affecting people today especially when it comes to the ecological and global worming problem around the world today. Many people today believe that the mass production of animals is one of the biggest contributors of this environmental problem today. I am trying to write in a very simple language for anybody to understand and from my own experience as a vegetarian for almost three decades. The first time I wrote about this topic was about 1982 and the difference between then and now is incredibly different and definitely more mature and concrete. I know from my own experience now what it takes to work and live as a vegetarian in the streets of a major city like New York. I first became a vegetarian for a religious reason I was studying Indian religions and philosophy to the point of teaching and instructing classes on Yoga. Throughout the years being a vegetarian and living the life of a vegetarian for almost 30 years it has given me more knowledge and understanding than books and religion would ever have given me. That is the main reason why I decided to write this book so I can share my experience with you and to unmask the truth about vegetarianism today. We must understand that being a vegetarian back then and one today is a whole different ball game. I believe that society is becoming more knowledgeable and more aware of their real role in the world today.

The method and approach that I will apply is the deductive method, arguing from the most basic principle to the most complex in order to try and understand the different standpoint taken, and to look at the matter without any bias and fanatism in favor of either vegetarianism or omnivorous or a mixed diet. The development of the argument will hopefully manifest itself intertwine and with both topics fully explained at the end. I will begin the argument by asking the question "What are the main reasons for a person to choose to be a vegetarian ".After a very careful and difficult study I have found that there are three main reasons that seems to cover the argument at hand, geared more toward the most complex of the two "Vegetarianism "remember that the whole of the argument is going to be a bit bias for we have to understand that the world is divided into Eastern and Western thoughts. Eastern and Western societies which are different in life style, religions, philosophical believes, and traditions being so different among themself that it's like night and day, we will deal with these issues in later chapters. The exposition is going to be geared more to the Western man and his daily living and daily needs, because I feel that the real difficulty is with the western man and the way he has become so dependent to the domestication of the animal kingdom and also to the vegetable kingdom for their personal need and survival. The three main reasons why people have chosen to become a vegetarian after being a meat eater (Omnivorous or mixed diet) all their life are, hygienic, humanitarian, and religious reasons. We will consider each of these separately, on their own merit and difficulties in order to try and understand such a difficult topic that's affecting the whole of society today.

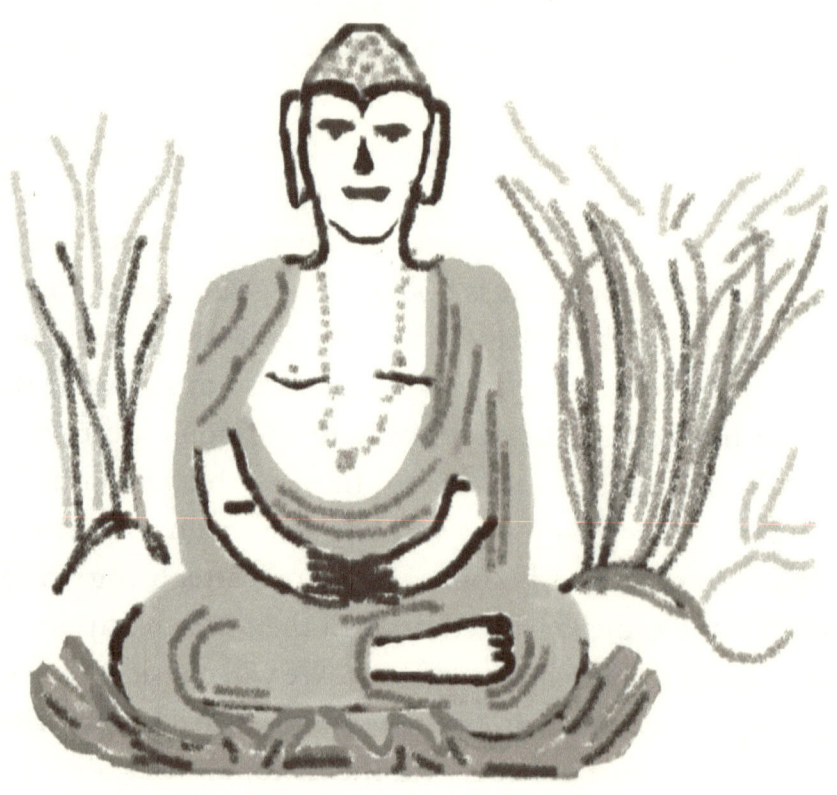

What is vegetarianism?

*N*ow let's start by defining what is vegetarianism and the way that it is being understood today.

A vegetarian is someone living on a diet of grains, pulses, (the edible seeds, peas, beans, lentils, and plants having pots) nuts, seeds, vegetables and fruits without the use of dairy products and eggs or anything that comes from the exploitation of animals like honey, wool, leather, and fur. Making him a person that is totally against the domestication and exploitation of animals. They are against anything that has to do with the cruelty of sentient beings the cruelty only extending itself to farmed animals and not to the whole of animals that are actually sacrifices every day. The ones that comes the closes to the ideal of a real "Vegetarians "are the ones that follow the vegan's way of diet because they are the only ones that only consume vegetables in their diets and don't have anything to do with the slaughter of animals and their by-products and really care of the exploitation of animals. The other groups that are involved in the use or consumption of these animal by—products such as eggs, milk, dairy products, honey, leather, wool, and fur do not really care for animals being exploited in an inhumane manner in the farming system and the ways that animals are being exploited today or they just don't understand the whole issue of being a vegetarian. We must understand that the problem is a lot more involved than just abstaining from flesh eating unless you are a vegetarian just for health reasons. This statement goes in accordance with the definition above of a vegetarian; the other groups are considered vegetarians simply because they do not eat meat but still enjoy using their by-products. A vegetarian does not eat any meat, poultry, game, fish, shellfish or crustacean, (which include, shrimps, and lobsters) or slaughter by-products. Like I mentioned before there are many groups, levels, and types of vegetarians all of them with their own motives and justifications some only care of cruelty to the animal kingdom while others go further and feel that it is also wrong to exploit the vegetable kingdom. While there are others that are vegetarians simply because of diet, and healthy reasons. Let's start by numerating the different types of diets with their definitions and their restrictions and motives.

TYPES OF VEGETARIANS

*T*hese are the different types of vegetarians throughout the world today

1) ovo-lacto vegetarian; eats eggs, milk, dairy products, all types of vegetables, fruits, nuts, and seed

2) Ovo vegetarian; eats eggs, all types of vegetables, fruits, nuts, and seeds.

3) lacto—vegetarian ; drinks milk, dairy products, all types of vegetables, fruits, nuts, and seeds

4) strict vegetarian or vegan ; a vegan excludes animal flesh(meat, poultry, fish, and seafood) animal products(leather, silk, wool, furs, lanolin, soap, and gelatin) a vegans diet consists totally of vegetables, fruits nuts, and seeds

5) fruitarian ; consists of raw fruits, and seeds, Examples are, pineapple, mangos, bananas, avocados, melons, berries, and the vegetable fruits such as, tomatoes, cucumbers olives dry nuts, hazelnuts, cashews, seeds, including sprouted seeds. Fruitarians do not eat cooked food.

Ovo-lacto vegetarian

An ovo-lacto vegetarian (also lacto-ovo vegetarian) is a vegetarian who does not eat beef, lamb, pork, poultry, fish, shellfish or animal flesh of any kind, but is willing to consume milk, dairy products, eggs, egg products, honey, and many even use furs, leathers, and wool. The terminology stems from the Latin lacto meaning "milk", ovo meaning "egg".

In the Western world lacto-ovo vegetarians are the most common type of vegetarian. Generally speaking, when one uses the term vegetarian a lacto-ovo vegetarian is assumed. Lacto-ovo vegetarianism is often motivated by ethics: it is thought by many followers of this diet that eggs and dairy are permitted because they don't involve slaughter of animals, but you see there is a lot of exploitation involved for they are not kept in their natural habitat and humane conditions and believe me they do not die of old age they are slaughter once they are useless for production. This exploitation is mainly only true in the modern food industry; there are many places in the world that produce milk and eggs in very humane conditions even though they are killed at the end of their productive life there are some places in India that they are not killed. Since eggs and milk are only produced by female chickens and cows, commercial food producers will often engage in the practice of sexing, whereby males are either slaughtered immediately (typical for chickens) or raised for meat (more common for cattle). Furthermore, both dairy cattle and egg-laying hens are slaughtered when they leave the period of peak productivity, which is typically much shorter than their natural lifespan.

Some ethically motivated lacto-ovo vegetarians may avoid fertilized eggs as well as caviar believing that both involve animal death. They may also avoid cheese that contains rennet and products that contain gelatin as there are animal products involved in their production.

Many Seventh-day Adventists are lacto-ovo vegetarians for over 130 years; Seventh-day Adventists have recommended a vegetarian diet which may include milk products and eggs their motives are for dietary reasons and not for animals well being.

Ovo-vegetarian

*O*vo vegetarianism is a type of vegetarianism which allows for the consumption of eggs; unlike lacto-ovo vegetarianism, no dairy products are permitted. Those who practice ovo vegetarianism are called ovo-vegetarians or "eggetarians." "Ovo" comes from the Latin word for egg.

Ethical motivations for excluding dairy products are based on issues with the industrial practices behind their production. Concerns include the practice of keeping a cow constantly pregnant in order for her to lactate and the slaughter of unwanted male calves, this is a process that is also used in the selection of hens, where they take the males for slaughter since they are useless for laying eggs. When the hens are also useless they also head to the slaughter house for meat so even if the meat is not consumed you are also responsible for the slaughter just for consuming eggs. Other concerns include the standard practice of separating the mother from her calf and denying the calf its natural source of milk. This contrasts with the industrial practices surrounding egg-laying hens, which produce eggs for human consumption without being fertilized. Ovo-vegetarians often prefer free-range eggs, particularly those produced by encaged hens. Carbon emissions associated with keeping hens are less than those associated with cattle, a factor significant to those practicing environmental vegetarianism.

Lacto vegetarian

A Lacto vegetarian (sometimes referred to as a lactarian) diet is a vegetarian diet which includes

Dairy products such as milk, cheese, yogurt, butter, cream, and kefir, but exclude eggs. The origin of "lacto" is the Latin word for milk (lac, lactise). Cheeses which include animal rennet and yogurts which contain gelatin are also avoided. The concept and practice of lacto-vegetarianism amongst a significant number of people comes from ancient India and was originally based on religious beliefs. Within Indian cultures this diet is often what is meant by the term "vegetarian". The greatest proportion of vegetarians, such as those in India or those in the area of the classical Mediterranean are lacto vegetarians and they don't usually kill the cows at the end of their productive life.

Lacto-vegetarians abstain from specifically eating eggs, fish, chickens, cows, sheep, pigs and sea animals. Eggs contain animal hormones including testosterone. Lacto vegetarianism may be adopted by vegetarians wishing to lower their dietary intake of cholesterol, since egg yolks, as well as dairy products, contain cholesterol. Unfertilized eggs contain a similar amount of cholesterol as fertilized eggs.

Lacto-vegetarian diets are popular with many followers of Eastern religious traditions such as Hinduism, Jainism and Buddhism. The core belief behind a lacto-vegetarian diet is the law of ahimsa, or non-violence. According to the Vedas (Hindu holy scriptures), all living beings are equally valued. Also, Hindus believe that one's personality is affected by the kind of food one consumes and eating flesh is considered bad for one's spiritual mental well-being and development, and the creation of negative Karma. It takes many more vegetables or plants to produce an equal amount of meat many more lives are destroyed and more suffering is caused when meat is used as food. In the case of Jainism, the vegetarian standards are even stricter. It only allows the consumption of fruit and leaves that can be taken from plants without causing their death. This further excludes from the diet vegetables like carrots, potatoes and peanuts. Although some suffering and pain is inevitably caused to other living beings to satisfy the human need for food, according to ahimsa, every effort should be made to minimize suffering. This is to avoid karmic consequences and show respect for God's creation. In this sense, wastage of food is considered a sin. Because all living beings are equally valued by God, vegetarian diet rooted in ahimsa is only one aspect of environmentally conscious living, relating to those beings affected by our need for food. Environmentalism and vegetarianism are often practiced together.

Vegans

O ut of all these different types of diets the vegan has the most complex of them all especially for the western man. We must remember that a vegetarian diet is not a natural diet for the western man that western society especially America is mostly based on an omnivorous (mixed diet) diet; we must understand that everything around us here in the west has in one way or another something to do with animal and their by-products. Western society has become almost totally dependent on animal and their by—products, the prove can be found in almost everything around us in medicine, glue, vehicles, electronic, furnishers, clothing, pastry, bread, and many, many more products that we are just not aware of for it has become so natural that it has been taken for granted the application of the use of these products. That's why it's very important for vegans to do their homework and investigate about such usage and read all labels. One thing that has to be remembered about labeling we must know how to read the scientific names for these animal products this happened to me and many of my friends many times looking for known words and not seeing anything thinking it was safe to use. There are many more complications about being a vegetarian (vegan) that will be dealt with in later chapters, such as the deficiencies of some very important vitamins, and the difficulty that the western people have in finding its substitutes. It must be understood that vegans will depend almost totally on dietary supplement in order to maintain proper health and this has a set of problem in its self that I will try to shed some light on. I have to stress again that vegans in order to carry some type of healthy life it is impossible without the total dependency of these supplements. Also it has to be understood that things get even more complicated when the motive for the individual to choose to be a vegetarian is the humanitarian reason, and how it's almost impossible to follow here in the Western part of the world. I will get more specific in later chapters for this is a very important and complex issue.

Fruitarian

*F*ruitarianism is the practice endorsed by people called fruitarians or fructarians of following a diet that comprises fruits, nuts and seeds, without animal products, and without vegetables and grains. Fruitarianism is a subset of veganism. Some people whose diet consists of 75% or more fruit consider themselves fruitarians.

Commonly the term "fruit" is used when referring to plant fruits that are sweet, fleshy and contain seeds within the plant fruit (for example, plums, apples, and oranges). However, there are other foods that are not typically considered to be fruits in a culinary sense but are botanically considered fruits, such as berries, bell peppers, eggplant, tomatoes, and cucumbers.

Some fruitarians will eat only what falls or would fall naturally from a plant or tree; that is: foods that can be harvested without killing the plant. These foods consist primarily of culinary fruits, nuts, and seeds. According to some fruitarians they eat only fallen fruit some do not eat grains believing it is unnatural to do so, and some fruitarians feel that it is improper for humans to eat seeds as they contain future plants. Some fruitarians use the botanical definitions of fruits and consume pulses, such as many beans and peas or legumes, or pulses and legumes. Some fruitarians believe fruitarianism was the original diet of humankind in the form of Adam and Eve based on Genesis 1:29. They believe that a return to an Eden-like paradise will require simple living and a holistic approach to health and diet. Some fruitarians wish, like Jains, to avoid killing anything, including plants and trees which are from the same family. There is a bit of a problem with this idea for Fruitarians for they should also avoid the use of any by-products made of wood like furnishers, an any houses made of wood, because we know what happens to trees when we do, we kill it just like killing any animal.

As a very extreme vegan diet, fruitarianism is highly restrictive, making nutritional adequacy almost impossible. It is reported that a fruitarian diet can cause deficiencies in calcium, protein, iron, zinc, vitamin D, most B vitamins (especially B12), and essential fatty acids. Additionally, it is reported that food restrictions in general may lead to hunger, cravings, food obsessions, social disruptions and social isolation. In children, growth and development are at risk. Nutritional problems include severe protein energy malnutrition, anemia and a wide range of vitamin and mineral deficiencies. Several children have died as the result of being fed fruitarian diets. As a result, children have been taken from parents feeding them fruitarian diets.

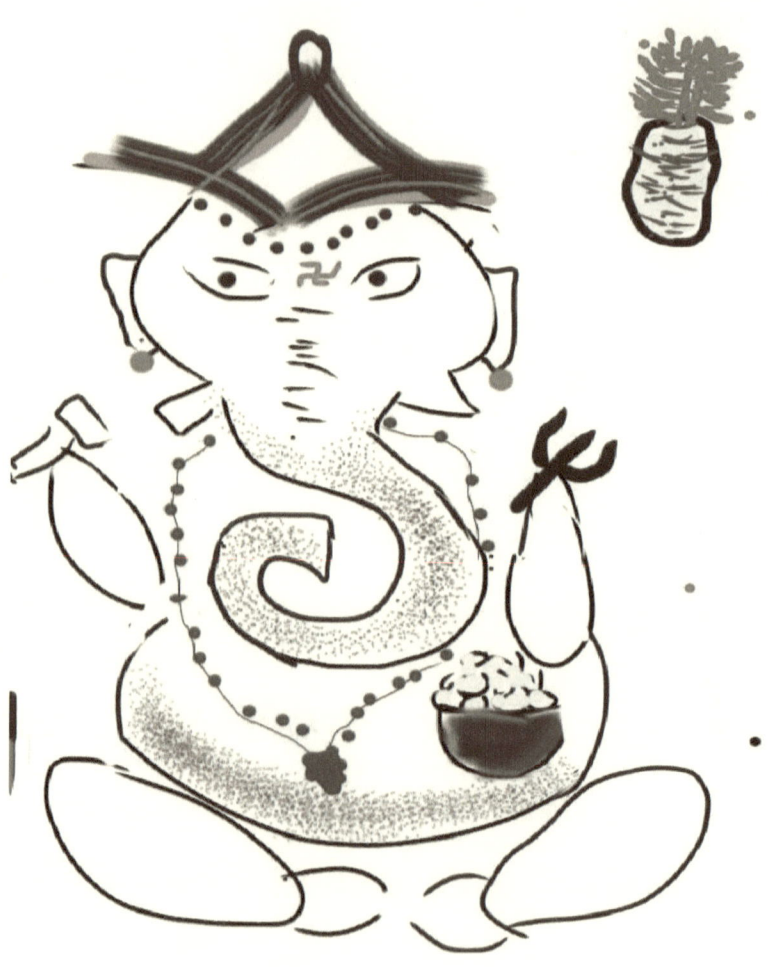

Stumbling Blocks

Many foods contain ingredients derived from the slaughter of animals that many vegetarians are not aware of and should really worry about finding out. Gelatin is hydrolyzed collagen, the main protein in animal connective tissue. Gelatin has historically been a prominent source of glue, musical instruments, embroidery, one of the main emulsions used in cosmetics, photographic film, the main coating given to medical capsule pills, and in the form of food including jelly, trifle, marshmallows, confectionery, low fat spread, dessert, and other daily products. Gelatin is made from animal ligaments, tendons, and bones extract which have been boiled in water. The term animal fat refers to carcass fat and may be present in a wide range of foods, including bread, pizzas, biscuits, cakes, pastries, margarines and the favorite for many restaurants. Suet and lard are types of animal fats. Certain food additives (E numbers) found in many foods may be derived from animal sources. Cheese is often made with rennet extracted from the stomach lining of slaughtered calves. Vegetarian cheese is made with rennet from a microbial source.

The Vegetarian Society has an information sheet listing ingredients and foods that should be avoided, which may be unsuitable for vegetarians. But it's always recommended for the person to do his own investigation for the simple fact that things around us are constantly changing either for good or worst for vegans.

Practices in catering and restaurants

Vegetarians dining out will expect work surfaces, cold cuts cutting machines, chopping boards, utensils, and all other kitchen equipment and facilities to be either kept separate from those used for non-vegetarian food preparation, or cleaned thoroughly before vegetarian food preparation. This is a major problem for vegans for it is very difficult for most restaurants to follow these guide lines.

Caterers should also ensure that fryers, grills and griddles used for preparing non-vegetarian products are thoroughly cleaned, we know that the total cleaning of this equipment back and forth is very difficult if not to say impossible. Fryers must be filled with fresh, uncontaminated oil before vegetarian food is cooked a process that is very costly and very troublesome and time consuming for these establishments and as much as they would like to keep them vegan safety especially on very busy skeduals it's almost impossible.

Vegans always recommend that caterers keep a separate set of utensils for the preparation and serving of vegetarian meals in order for them to consume any food in their establishment. The majority of vegans will not eat anything in restaurants that sell animal product because of this very difficult problem they run the risk of getting something unclean. I have a family member that goes around with his own pots and pans when he travels in order to maintain some control of what he consumes. We must try to understand that in the western part of world most restaurants and food establishments in major cities, and especially in small cities and towns don't even know about vegans, and are just set up for meat consumption. For a person to be a vegan and have a busy scheduled job, has a very difficult task ahead of him no matter where you go for food you have to be very careful and I guaranteed that it is almost impossible to eat clean and healthy under these condition this I speak out my own experience of working and living in a major city and having to go without eating because I could not find any vegetarian food around, this I know for I have been a vegetarian for over 25 years and had to suffer and endure to the point of sacrificing my health and even having to go hungry at times.

From all this that was said it can be concluded that the vegan diet is not the healthiest or the easiest of the two diets. It is not the healthiest because of the difficulty in balancing the physical needs for every person under all circumstances. Once a very famous Sage said "all extremes should be avoided ", anything that we bring to an extreme will eventually cause harm, this principal can be applied to everything in life. For example food is very good for the body but if we eat too much of it, it will cause obesity and harm us eventually, than with the same token if we do not eat enough food we will lose too much weight become anemic and in turn harm us. This same principle applied to diet will have the same results, any diet whether carnivorous, vegan, or fruitarian that is taken to the extreme will become a health issue for the individual abusing their diet for whatever reason they have, let it be hygienic, humanitarian, or religious. People who have been known to have a more than 90% meat diet because of where they live have been known to have a very short life span. While looking to the other extreme people who are very strict vegetarians wind up becoming anemic and having real health issues. I do not mean to imply by all this that it is not possible to maintain health in a strict vegetarian diet, but I do maintain that it is not possible for everybody to do so under all circumstances. And it becomes even more difficult when the reason for choosing a vegan way of live is the humanitarian idea. To take a person accustomed to an ordinary mixed diet, and start him on a strict vegetarian diet and his normal life at the same time is rarely satisfactory, especially if that person is engaged in a strenuous and stressful life style and occupation like myself, or has difficulties in getting meat substitutes in his daily walk of life. This is too often done by people every day and it is a very unwise method of procedure. The main reason for this book is to unmask all the misconceptions about vegetarianism and to try to help people to become one not through emotion but through facts and a scientific attitude, and to know all the difficulties one will face in this very important and most difficult decision. It must be understood that a decision about becoming a vegan is a decision that will affect the whole of your life not just your diet, diet being just fifty % of your new life style and difficulty in life, and believe me I am not just being negative, but a realize, for I am speaking from my very own experience.

Three main reasons for choosing a vegetarian Diet

*I*n this very important chapter we will discuss the main reasons for a person that is already a vegetarian, and one who is just choosing to be one to hopefully understand what he is involved in. I will unmask the truth about the reasons why a person chooses to be a vegetarian and try to bypass all the emotional miss understanding that is usually involved in making such an important decision in a person's life. This decision is usually based on emotions or simply because some famous person or some religious believe hundreds or even thousands of years old said it was all right. I will base my facts on new medical and scientific facts that should help in such an important decision. The three main reasons that are going to be discussed in this chapter should cover the whole issue of why to be a vegetarian today.

Hygienic, Diet

ygienic; The science of health and its maintenance

Diet; A limited or special selection of food and drink chosen or prescribed to promote health.

This is one of the reasons for a person to be or to become a vegetarian today mostly basing their reasons that man is and has always been a vegetarian animal and that this diet should be taken by everybody today without exceptions. Like I stated before this is a very emotional topic today and because of lack of understanding many people are venturing into something that they have very limited understanding about, and are going into it just by emotions and being dragged into it by people that don't have a clue about it. I have seen this happen so many times in spiritual groups and yoga schools that base themselves on traditions and not medical facts. We have to understand that something like diet is not like fashion or what is the best car this is something that if we make the wrong choice it could mean the difference between a healthy life or one with irreversible damages even death.

Once a very famous doctor wrote something so true that will shed some light to the subject at hand, of the best and most appropriate diet for every individual. Most people seem to think ; he said, that although there is an infinite variety about the way we look on the outside, there are, small, big, skinny, fat, strong, weak, healthy, sickly, and people with very serious health issues to name a few, all with totally different needs. People seem to believe that our insides are just a sealed pattern that all of us just have organs, blood, bones, muscles, and nerves and that we are all alike inside. He said, that in his office he has a large collection of x—ray photographs and that he can recognize his different patients by the portraits of their insides just as he could by the photographs of their faces. If there is so much difference in their internal appearance must there not be an equal difference in their internal needs? The point that I am trying to make is that if, just as there are different people with different physiological needs there should be different diets according to their needs. The point that I am trying to get across and want people to understand is that diets not only should be different because of the physiology of the person, but also because of their daily activities and also because of their geographical locations. With all this being said what I am saying and trying to bring to light is the complexity of the physical body and its daily needs.

Are vegetarian diets healthful?

Vegetarian diets can be healthful and nutritionally sound if they're carefully planned individually, with this I am trying to say we are all different inside and have different dietary needs. However, a vegetarian diet can be unhealthy if it contains too many calories and/or saturated fat and not enough important nutrients and essential vitamins in their complete diet, we will mention some of the most important ones complete with their resources.

Nutrients and Vitamins to consider in a basic vegetarian diet.

Dietary supplements

In the United States, a dietary supplement is defined as a product that is intended to supplement the diet and contains any of the following dietary ingredients: vitamins, minerals, herbs, some botanical ingredients, and amino acids. It comes as a concentrate, metabolite, constituent, extract, or a combination of two or more mentioned. They come in many forms such as pills, capsules, tablets, liquid form, and powder. Not represented for use as a conventional food or as the sole item of a meal or diet they must be taken as a food supplement.

Dietary supplements are used for different purposes especially to supply needs that one's daily diet is not covering effectively. However, vitamin detractors, for instance, have claimed supplements can be harmful and have more cons than pros. Nevertheless, many specialists defend their use and support it with vast evidence. They also insist that nutritional deficiency is hard to avoid in times when lifestyles are extremely busy and consumption of fast food is high or the change of an omnivore diet to a vegan diet.

All dietary supplement manufacturers have to ensure by June 2010 that production of dietary supplements complies with current good manufacturing practices, and are manufactured with "controls that result in a consistent product free of contamination, with accurate labeling. In addition, the industry is now required to report to the FDA all serious dietary supplement related adverse events after they happen of course and the damage to the consumer has been done. The new rules have been criticized, however, with skeptics arguing lack of FDA resources, loopholes, and an exception on quality assurance for raw material suppliers (with the burden placed on manufacturers) this will lead to continued quality problems for the consumer for there is no assurance of quality control, or if the supplement even has what the label states it has and the inability of the FDA or the manufactures to test the raw material suppliers. There's also concern that supplement manufacturers and retailers will hide behind the new regulations given by the FDA. Prior to the rule supplements have had major quality problems, and the number of FDA investigators has declined making it more difficult in making sure that the manufacturers are kept honest and to comply with their labeling claim. This has been the cause for many Law suits against manufacturing companies, from physical damages caused to consumers from false claims due to lack of real testing of their products, and no pressure from FDA department. This is the main reason why I am writing about dietary supplement in order to unmask the truth for the vegetarian communities about supplements and how damaging it could be to them since they are so dependent on them.

If a dietary supplement claims to cure, mitigate, or treat a disease, it would be considered an unauthorized and in violation of the applicable regulations and statutes.

It is illegal to market a dietary supplement product as a treatment or cure for a specific disease or condition?

A product sold as a dietary supplement and promoted on its label or in labeling as a treatment, prevention or cure for a specific disease or condition would be considered an unapproved and thus illegal drug and still many manufactures make claims about their products on labels and TV. To maintain the product's status as a dietary supplement, the label and labeling must be consistent with the provisions in the Dietary Supplement Health and Education Act.

Dietary supplements are permitted to make structure/function claims. These are broad claims that the product can support the structure or function of the body. (The FDA must be notified of these claims within 30 days of their first use, and there is a requirement that these claims be substantiated. In reality, misleading claims about supplements are common even in today's market due to government's inability to follow up.

The department of the USA, (DSHEA) says by law, the manufacturer is responsible for ensuring that its dietary supplement products are safe before they are marketed. Unlike drug products that must be proven safe and effective for their intended use before marketing, there are no provisions in the law for FDA to "approve" dietary supplements for labeling, safety or effectiveness before they reach the consumer.

Do manufacturers or distributors of dietary supplements have to tell FDA or consumers what evidence they have about their product's safety or what evidence they have to back up the claims they are marketing for?

No, except for rules described above that govern new dietary ingredients, there is no provision under any law or regulation that FDA enforces that requires a firm to disclose to FDA or consumers the information they have about the safety or purported benefits of their dietary supplement products, that's why there has been many Law suits against supplement firms like I mentioned above. Likewise, there is no prohibition against them making this information available either to FDA or to their customers. It is up to each firm to set its own policy on disclosure of such information putting the real burden on the consumer on having to trust these companies with their health for as I mentioned above that groups such as vegans and fruitarians have to depend almost totally on these supplements in order to gain some vitamins that are not found in vegetables. The lack of these very important vitamins and minerals in their diets and especially in their kids can be devastating. The real burden is that the consumer might think that he is getting something that he is not and when he comes to realize it the damage is already done.

Because dietary supplements are under the umbrella of foods, they don't have to say anything about their products that they don't want the consumers to know and the FDA does not have to know either.

As I stated above, that especially for people living the vegetarian diet (especially for vegans), who become totally dependent to supplements in order to maintain health they should be extremely careful in choosing dietary supplements for themselves and especially for your young ones, for this can cause permanent damage to your health, and especially to your young kids that need all their nutrient and vitamins in order to have a healthy development. This is why I am trying to unmask the truth about dietary supplements and show how extremely important it is to have a real understanding about them. It is extremely important for vegetarians to do their homework when it comes to supplement companies and what they claim in their labels always remembering that most supplements don't come from natural and clean resources anyway. Please try to find a company you feel comfortable with and always check your self and especially your kids. Always remember that young kids don't have the luxury that some adults have when it comes to the accumulation of vitamin B12 in their liver damages will be very fast and in most cases permanent.

The real problem with dietary supplements today.

The failure to control quality is one reason why the safety of dietary supplements cannot be assured.

Recent polls have shown that up to 64% of Americans take at least one dietary supplement a day, and with a high percentage of them taking more than one supplement at the sometime. Combining a number of supplements from different manufactures is heading for big problems. Manufacturers do not get together discussing how their formulas can integrate with each other's products they don't even label warnings about the interactions of products and the side effects that they can cause simply because it is not in their best of interest. Sadly, it is common practice for manufacturers to include a considerable amount of additional ingredients, in order to make their products more attractive, and to make their formula stand out amongst many competitors. Multiple products taking this "add-on" approach can easily lead to excessive and potentially problematic nutrient intakes because they are never tested for side effects before getting to the consumer.

One of the main problems with supplements is that the manufacturer decides if a product is safe for consumers. Government testing and approval is not required. In fact, a manufacturer is not even required to register their product with the US Food and Drug Administration unless a new dietary ingredient is used.

In this competitive industry, manufacturers can push the limit trying to find a combination of supplements that offer the most benefits with an acceptable amount of risk to you the consumer. They determine what mixtures of supplements can be used, how much of each supplement is added and what is an acceptable amount with little or no testing, and what is a safe amount for consumers. If injuries occur due to usage or over usage, the FDA must prove the product unreasonably harmful before taking action. The Food and Drug Administration (FDA) regulates dietary supplements. While dietary supplement manufacturers are responsible for the safety of their products, they do not need to get government approval before producing or selling their products. FDA is not responsible for determining the efficacy of dietary supplements. The law specifies certain conditions under which FDA can take action to remove a dietary supplement from the market based on evidence that it presents a significant or unreasonable risk or is otherwise adulterated of course by this time the damage has been done to some ignorant consumer. The advertising of dietary supplements is regulated by the Federal Trade Commission (FTC).

The FDA does not analyze dietary supplements before they are sold to consumers. The manufacturer is responsible for ensuring that the "Supplement Facts" label and ingredient list are accurate, that the dietary ingredients are safe, and that the content matches the amount declared on the manufactures labeling. This is why there are so many Law Suits against manufactures today. There are many Law firms that make millions on these types of Law suits each year.

Additional problem with dietary supplements

A lack of knowledge about long-term effects of using supplements is also a major problem. There is simply not enough testing to know what damage a product can cause to the body after long term use.

Another of the chief problems with supplements is that people often use them without a physician's knowledge or an adequate understanding of how the supplements change the body. If you want to lose weight or increase your endurance, you can find a few supplements that are suppose to help and take them. However, you may be unaware that those very supplements could be causing your body much more harm than good. Education is the key, but how many of the millions of people regularly using supplements actually understand the effects they have on the body or the side effects they can cause? If a preexisting medical condition exists, or if other supplements or drugs (over-the-counter or prescription) are also taken, the risks for side effects can increase greatly.

Some people use dietary supplements rather than seeking professional medical treatment when needed, although those supplements may not actually be providing any benefits. This is considered another problem with supplements.

Multivitamins

*T*he next topic multivitamins that I will write about, because of their categorization as a dietary supplement by the Food and Drug Administration (FDA), most multivitamins sold in the U.S. are not required to undergo the rigorous testing procedures typical of pharmaceutical drugs. They also fall under the same rules and regulations of dietary supplements and with that also comes all the problems and difficulties written about dietary supplements in the last chapter.

A multivitamin is a preparation intended to supplement a human diet with vitamins, dietary minerals and other nutritional elements. Such preparations are available in the form of tablets, capsules, pastilles, powders, liquids and inject able formulations. Other than inject able formulations, which are only available and administered under medical supervision, multivitamins are recognized by the Codex Alimentarius Commission (the United Nations' authority on food standards) as a category of food. Multivitamin supplements are commonly provided in combination with minerals. A multivitamin/mineral supplement is defined in the United States as a supplement containing 3 or more vitamins and minerals that does not include herbs, hormones, or drugs, where each vitamin and mineral is included at a dose below the tolerable upper level, as determined by the Food and Drug Board, and does not present a risk of adverse health effects. The terms multivitamin and multimineral are often used interchangeably. There is no scientific definition for either. Linguistically, the terms are compounded words of which meaning can be derived in that capacity.

In 2006 the National Institutes of Health convened an expert panel to examine the available evidence on nutrient supplements. This review concluded that "Most of the studies we examined do not provide strong evidence for beneficial health-related effects of supplements taken singly, in pairs, or in combinations of three or more." They noted that multivitamins could provide health benefits to some groups of people, such as postmenopausal women, but that there was "disturbing evidence of risk" in other groups, such as smokers. The panel's report concluded that the "present evidence is insufficient to recommend either for or against the use of Multivitamin/Mineral Supplements by the American public to prevent chronic disease. Prenatal vitamins contain higher levels of iron and folic acid, compared with typical multivitamins

However, some multivitamins contain very high doses of one or several vitamins or minerals, or are specifically intended to treat, cure, or prevent disease, and therefore require a prescription or medicinal license in the U.S. Since such drugs contain no new substances, they do not require the same testing as would be required by a New Drug Application, but were allowed on the market as drugs due to the Drug Efficacy Study Implementation program.

Protein

*P*lant proteins alone can provide enough of the essential and non-essential amino acids, as long as sources of dietary protein are varied and caloric intake is high enough to meet energy needs.

Whole grains, legumes, vegetables, seeds and nuts all contain both essential and non-essential amino acids.

Soy protein can be your sole protein source if you choose. Vegetarians do not have any problem in acquisition of proteins (including vegans)

Iron

Vegetarians may have a greater risk of iron deficiency than non vegetarians. The richest sources of iron are red meat, liver and egg yolk—all high in cholesterol. However, dried beans, spinach, enriched products, brewer's yeast and dried fruits are all good plant sources of iron where available.

Sea vegetables like nori, wakame, and dulse are very high in iron. Less exotic but still good options are iron-fortified breakfast cereals, legumes (chickpeas, lentils, and baked beans), soybeans and tofu, dried fruit (raisins and figs), pumpkin seeds, broccoli, and blackstrap molasses. Eating these foods along with a food high in vitamin C (citrus fruits and juices, tomatoes, and broccoli) will help you to absorb the iron better.

Girls need to be particularly concerned about getting adequate iron because some iron is lost during menstruation. Some girls who are vegetarians may not get adequate iron from vegetable sources and they may require a daily supplement

Vitamin B-12

*T*his comes naturally only from animal sources. Vegans need a reliable source of vitamin B-12. It can be found in some fortified (not enriched) breakfast cereals, fortified soy beverages, fortified breakfast bars (fortified means that it is added to the food and not a natural part of it. I make a point of this because many of my friends were confused and thought that vitamin B12 was part of the food that was being fortified thinking that the soy beans products were B12 enriched. That's why it's very important to check, read, and understand the labels to see exactly what you are taking. We must understand that this is the most complex and important of all the vitamins I will dedicate a whole chapter to this vitamin because of its importance to vegetarians and also to non-vegetarians.

Vitamin D

People need vitamin D to get calcium into our bones. Your body manufactures vitamin D when your skin is exposed to sunlight. Cow's milk is top on the list for food sources of this vitamin. Vegans can try fortified soy milk and fortified breakfast cereals. Some people may need a supplement that includes vitamin D, especially during the winter months. Everyone should have some exposure to the sun to help the body produce vitamin D.

Calcium

*M*ilk and yogurt are tops if you're eating dairy products—although vegetarians will want to look for yogurt that does not contain the meat by-product gelatin. Tofu, fortified soy milk, calcium-fortified orange juice, green leafy vegetables, and dried figs are also excellent ways for vegetarians (and vegans) to get calcium. Remember that as a teen you're building up your bones for the rest of your life, and whatever damages are done while growing up will be yours for life.

Because women have a greater risk for getting osteoporosis (weak bones) as adults, it's particularly important for girls to make sure they get enough calcium. Again, taking a supplement may be necessary to ensure this.

Zinc

Zinc is needed for growth and development. Good plant sources include grains, nuts and legumes. Shellfish are an excellent source of zinc. Take care to select supplements containing no more than 15-18 mg zinc. Supplements containing 50 mg or more may lower HDL ("good") cholesterol in some people.

Are These Diets healthy and safe for Teens and babies?

*Y*es it has been proven that a vegetarian diet could be healthy to teens and babies, but a lot more complicated than a mixed diet (omnivorous) for in mixed diets teens and babies always get all the right nutrients without the needs of supplements and don't have to worry about all the social problems it brings. Especially for vegan kids it becomes healthy and emotionally extremely difficult, but not impossible of course. Parents have to be more aware of their kid's diet and social interactions with friends, and especially at school because almost all schools in western societies are geared to a omnivorous way of live not only in the food they serve but in everything else. We as parents don't have a clue how difficult it is to take a kid let's say five years old and over after eating meat, and wearing leather shoes, sneakers, fashion belts, glue for school, toys containing animal products, and especially fast food. It should take some special dealing from their parents in helping them understand to deal with their parent's new way of living. Like I said before that this is not only a dietary problem but something that takes over your whole life and it all depends how far you're willing to go. I believe that teens and younger kids are the ones that really have to sacrifice their lives, and to understand why they are different than most of their friends, so the burden for parents is not a walk in the park. In the past, choosing not to eat meat or animal-based foods was considered unusual in the United States. Times and attitudes have changed dramatically. There are about 4 million vegetarians in the USA alone, Vegetarians are still a minority in the United States, but are a large and growing one which gives me more reason to write this book. The American Dietetic Association (ADA) has officially endorsed vegetarianism, stating "appropriately planned vegetarian diets, including total vegetarian or vegan diets, are healthful, and nutritionally adequate if properly understood. Remember this has nothing to do with the social problem and difficulties in finding meat substitute this is only talking in a dietary sense and if everything is right.

If you and your family are choosing a vegetarian diet the most important thing you can do is to educate yourself on what exactly you're getting involved in for the well being of you and your family. That's why the ADA says that a vegetarian diet needs to be "appropriately planned." Simply dropping certain foods from your diet isn't the way to go if you're interested in maintaining good health, a high energy level, and strong muscles and bones. Remembering that now your diet is going to be very dependent on supplements in order to have a healthy live. We must remember that we don't know the side effects of all supplements and understand that many of them are not from natural sources I gave a good explanation about them in earlier chapters.

If meat, fish, dairy products, and/or eggs are not going to be part of your diet, you'll need to know how to get enough of these nutrients, or you may need to take a daily multiple vitamin and mineral supplement which in reality makes the whole process totally unnatural.

Fat, Calories, and Fiber

*I*n addition to vitamins and minerals, vegetarians need to keep an eye on their total intake of calories and fat. Vegetarian diets tend to be high in fiber and low in fat and calories. That may be good for people who need to lose weight or lower their cholesterol but it can be a problem for kids and teens who are still growing and people who are already at a healthy weight. One thing that I find about most vegans is that they tend to over eat because they stopped the consumption of meat in their diets, and this precedence is not very healthy.

Some vegetarians (especially vegans) may not get enough omega-3 fatty acids. Omega-3 fats are good for heart health and are found in fish and eggs. Some products, such as soy milk and breakfast bars, are fortified with Docosahexaenoic acid (DHA), an omega-3 fatty acid you have to read the labels and hope that they are accurate.

Diets that are high in fiber tend to be more filling, and as a result strict vegetarians may feel full before they've eaten enough calories to keep their bodies healthy and strong.

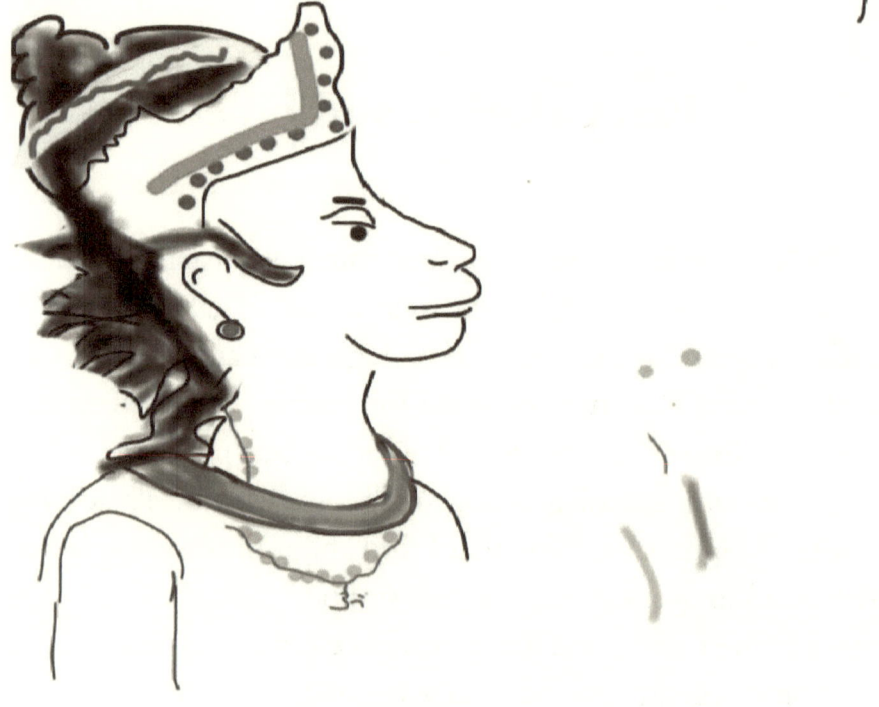

Humanitarian

*T*he question of vegetarianism from the humanitarian standpoint is also an extremely complex topic, and not nearly as simple as its advocates would have you believe. There are two main reasons for a person to chose to be a vegetarian because of humane reasons, they are, the eco-system problem around the world, and the inhumane slaughter of animals in modern farming system stating that it is wrong and inhumane to kill sentient being. The whole issue must depend on our attitude and understanding when it comes to the domestication and the exploitation of animals in the world today. Was it wrong for man to domesticate them? Was it essential for our ancestors in order to survive to domesticate them? Are domestic animals essential to civilization today? If we admit that the domestication and the exploitation of the animal kingdom is morally wrong, is it also wrong when it comes to the vegetable or plant kingdom which also have been domesticated and exploited by man with very good results in the help with world hunger and the total increase of humanity throughout the world. I believe that without the domestication and exploitation of these kingdoms there would not be any humanity as we have today for if man would have continued to feed themselves from the wild we would problebly be extinct or just a few hundred of us in existent and the world would still be in the dark ages and not as advanced as we are today. So you see the domestication of this kingdom by our ancestor was very necessary in order for man to be where he is today. If we admit that the exploitation of one natural kingdom over another is fundamentally and morally wrong, people of sensitive conscious will feel it incumbent upon them to reframe from the participation in their exploitation. But the exploitation consists much more then flesh eating; it involves the whole of sacrificing the live of living things by the selfish and neglectful behavior of humans we will have to find a line of demarcation and choose how far we are willing to go and agree what has to be sacrificed and what should be saved. Let's start now by trying to understand animals and what composes the animal kingdom.

Animals

Animals are a major group of mostly multicellular, eukaryotic organism of the kingdom Animalia or Metazoa. With the ability to move and obtain food, with specialized sense organs, and sexual reproduction organs. Most animals are motile, meaning they can move spontaneously and independently.

Etymology

The word "animal" comes from the Latin word *animal* (meaning *with soul*, from *anima*, soul). In everyday usage, the word usually refers to non-human animals. Frequently only closer relatives of humans such as vertebrates or mammals are meant in its use. The biological definition of the word refers to all members of the Kingdom Animalia, encompassing creatures ranging from insects to humans.

Characteristics

Animals have several characteristics that set them apart from other living things. Animals are multicellular which separates them from bacteria and most protists. They generally digest food in an internal chamber, which separates them from plants and algae. They are also distinguished from plants, algae, and fungi by lacking rigid cell walls. In most animals, embroil pass through a blastula stages, which is a characteristic exclusive to animals.

All animals are heterotrophs, meaning that they feed directly or indirectly on other living things. They are often further subdivided into groups such as carnivores, herbivores, omnivores, and parasites. I will go into the explanation of each of the different groups of animals so that we can see exactly what we mean by animals, that animals are not just the ones we see in farms and that the exploitation of man to the animal kingdom is not just these farm animals. From this we will also gather exactly where we fit in the animal kingdom

Carnivore

Carnvore (pronounced /ˈkɑrnɪvɔːr/), meaning 'meat eater' (Latin *carne* meaning 'flesh' and *vorare* meaning 'to devour'), is an organism that derives its energy and nutrient requirements from a diet consisting mainly or exclusively of animal tissue, whether through predation or scavenging. Animals that depend solely on animal flesh for their nutrient requirements are considered obligate carnivores while those that also consume non-animal food are considered facultative carnivores. Omnivorous also consume both animal and non-animal food, and apart from the more general definition, there is no clearly defined ratio of plant to animal material that would distinguish a carnivore from an omnivore, or an omnivore from a herbivore, for that matter. A carnivore that sits at the top of the food chain is an apex predator.

Plants that capture and digest insects are called carnivorous plants. Similarly fungi that capture microscopic animals are often called carnivorous fungi.

Obligate or true carnivores depend solely on the nutrients found in animal flesh for their survival. While they may consume small amounts of plant material, they lack the physiology required for the efficient digestion of vegetable matter and, in fact, some carnivorous mammals eat vegetation specifically as an emetic. The domestic cat is a prime example of an obligate carnivore, as are all of the other felids

Herbivores

*H*erbivores are animal that are adapted to eat plants. Herbivore is a form of predation in which an organism consumes principally autographs such as plants, algae and photosynthesizing bacteria. More generally, organisms that feed on autographs in general are known as primary consumers.

By definition, many fungi, some bacteria, many animals, some protists and a small number of parasitic plants might be considered herbivores. However, *herbivore* generally refers to animals eating plants.

Herbivores form an important link in the food chain as they consume plants in order to receive the carbohydrates produced by a plant from photosynthesis. Carnivorous in turn consume herbivores for the same reason, while omnivorous can obtain their nutrients from either plants or herbivores. Due to an herbivore's ability to survive solely on tough and fibrous plant matter, they are termed the primary consumers in the food cycle or food chain.

Herbivores are limited in their feeding ability by either time or resources. Animals that are time limited, meaning they have a limited amount of time to consume the food they need, use a feeding strategy of grazing and browsing, while those animals that are resource limited, meaning that they are limited in the type of food they eat, use a selective feeding strategy. Grazers/browsers tend to be either very large herbivores that need to consume a lot of food in order to maintain their metabolism, or herbivores that have a very short amount of time to eat as much as possible before reproducing, like many generalist insects.

Omnivores

Omnivore(from Latin: Omni all, everything; to devour) are species that eats both plants and animals as their primary food source. They are opportunistic, general feeders not specifically adapted to eat and digest either meat or plant material primarily. Pigs are one well-known example of an omnivore. Crows are another example of an omnivore that many people see every day. Humans are regarded as omnivores. Although the term omnivore literally means eater of everything, omnivores other than humans cannot really eat "everything" that other animals eat; they can only eat things that are at least moderately easy to get and still at least moderately nutritious. For example, most of them cannot live by grazing and easy to get, but not nutritious enough, nor can they eat some hard-shelled animals or successfully hunt large or fast prey nutritious, but too hard to get.

Although there are cases of herbivores eating meat matter, as well as examples of carnivores eating plants, the classification refers to the adaptations and main food source of the species in general, so these exceptions do not make either individual animals or the species as whole omnivores.

Most bear's species are considered omnivores, but individuals' diets can range from almost exclusively herbivorous to almost exclusively carnivorous, depending on what food sources are available locally and seasonally. Polar bears are classified as carnivores while pandas are classified as herbivores, although giant pandas will eat some meat (insects) from time to time, and polar bears will sometimes eat plants (kelp) but neither is a significant part of their diet. Species considered omnivorous.

Various mammals are omnivorous by nature, such as pigs, badgers, bears, coatis, hedgehogs, opossums, skunks, sloths, squirrels, raccoons, chipmunks, mice and rats. Also some primates are omnivorous including humans and chimpanzees. Various birds are omnivorous, whose diet varies from berries and nectar to insects, worms, fish, and small rodents; examples include cassowary, chickens, and crows and related In addition, some lizards, turtles, fish, such as piranhas, and invertebrates are also omnivorous.

Parasite

A parasite is an organism that lives on or inside another organism to the detriment of the host organism.

Parasitism is a type of symbiotic relationship between organisms of different species where one organism, the parasite, benefits at the expense of the hosts.

In general, parasites are much smaller than their host, show a high degree of specialization and are their mode of life, and reproduce more quickly and in greater numbers than their hosts. Classic examples of parasitism include interactions between vertebrate's hosts and diverse animals such as tapeworms, flukes, and fleas. Parasitism is differentiated from parasitoidism, a relationship in which the host is always killed by the parasite such as moths, butterflies, ants, flies and others. Parasites increase their fitness by exploiting hosts for food, habitat and dispersal.

Although the concept of parasitism applies unambiguously to many cases in nature, it is best considered part of a continuum of types of interaction between species, rather than an exclusive category. Particular interactions between species may satisfy some but not all parts of the definition. In many cases, it is difficult to demonstrate that the host is harmed. In others, there may be no apparent specialization on the part of the parasite, or the interaction between the organisms may be short-lived. In medicine, only eukaryotic organisms are considered parasites, with the exclusion of bacteria and viruses. Some branches of biology, however, regard members of these groups as parasitic.

Humanitarianism explained

*T*he suffering and cruelty inflicted upon farmed animals is a major cause for concern and a strong motivation for many vegans. Many people are becoming increasingly aware of the animal welfare concerns surrounding food production, particularly in intensive farming systems. However, the welfare of farmed animals during their lifetimes is not the only reason why vegans choose not to consume or use animal products.

There is strong evidence from behavioral studies that farmed animals such as pigs, chickens, ducks, turkeys, cows, sheep and fish are sentient beings with individual needs and preferences in life. The mass production and killing of these animals does not recognize this individual need of these animals. Anyone who has spent time with a companion animal knows that they have complex emotions and yet farmed animals are no different in this respect from dogs and cats.

Killing is an inherent and unavoidable part of farming animals for food. Of course animals are killed for meat, but many people are unaware that this is equally true of egg and milk production. Millions of male chicks and calves are killed each year as 'by-products' of the egg and milk industries, considered worthless since they cannot produce milk or eggs. The dairy cows and egg-laying hens themselves are killed at a fraction of their natural lifespan, when they become too worn out to produce enough milk or eggs to be profitable. Simply buying 'higher-welfare' animal products cannot change these facts.

The idea that these animals' pigs, cows, chickens, turkeys, ducks, sheep's, and fish are sentient beings, there should be major concern about their welfare. Should not this concern be also extended to the rest of the animal kingdom and not just to the ones that we eat or the ones that are farmed or have been already domesticated? I think that we should look further and see where the real cruelty and maybe senseless killing is being done, it is being done to the animals that are not domesticated and are being slaughtered for the simple reason that they are invading our environment which also is there environment and are there to live and survive. From the definition above we should be able to understand that the animal kingdom is very complex and extensive and they are all sentient beings with complex emotions and individual needs, if we look carefully we can see that the farmed animals are not the smartest or most functional of animals in the animal kingdom. So do we really have the right to pick and choose which animals to care for and let the cruelty continue with the rest of them.

We know of some Eastern school that teach a very strict principal when it comes to animal killing and exploitation, Jain priests carry a very soft broom with them and gently sweep the path before them as they walk lest they should accidently tread on some creepy creature and take its live. Some also walk around with a mask in order not to kill millions of animals that we always kill simply by breathing. We also know of some Indian Ascetics that refuse to remove maggots from their sores, even going to the length of replacing them when they fell off.

You see these principals have never taken good in the west, UK, America, and Europe. So you see when we talk about humanitarian motive for not eating meat, eggs, milk, honey, and any animal by-product we have to analyze to what extent it's a logical and a healthy decision making, and not a fad or extremely emotional decision. The idea that I am trying to make is that for a person to become a vegan because of dietary reasons saying that a vegetarian diet is healthier than a meat based diet is a matter of opinion that only affects the individual, but when people say that they are vegans because of the cruelty to animal and only worry about a handful of animals is not as easy and clear as people really believe it to be. I believe that no matter how much we try some animals will be sacrificed in order for us to live our daily lives whether intentional or unintentional, unless we are willing to sacrifice our way of life as we know it, and walk around with a soft broom and mask in order not to kill any of our animal friends. I don't believe that civilization today can go on without the sacrifice of some of the animal

Kingdom, whether it be mammals, fish, bees, fowls, or insects. For even doing the most basic things like, walking, breathing, driving a car, drinking water, to name a few some sentient being will be sacrificed. Someone asks; Will you kindly explain why, if you think it wrong to kill a pig, cow or a chicken for food, but it's ok to kill a water bug, mice, ants, flies, mosquitoes, flees, bed bugs, lice, rats, and smaller sentient beings that we just don't care about, simply with the reason that they are invading our space and threatening our surrounding trying to survive themselves. These animals are being slaughtered by the millions simply because of our own selfish reasons and nobody seems to care when you go to the super market go to the pest control isle and see the weapons used for the real murder and slaughter done to the animal kingdom. The question of right and wrong are somewhat mixed on this subject, the idea should be that all animals should be treated with the same love and care, all of life has its purpose in the web of life. If we look at nature everything is feeding off of something in order to survive the big problem right now is that man who is at the top of the food chain has to find a way to balance the whole ecology of the world and I believe and trust that humanity is heading in the right direction there are many people that really are worried and concerned about nature and the damage that we as humans are doing. We must understand that if it is wrong to kill all animals than it is wrong to live at all, you must understand that in the air that we breath and the water that we drink, there are millions of animals that are being instantly destroyed, they are called (infusorians, animalcule) yes they are living moving being as much as cows, pigs, chickens, bugs, ants, bees, and most animals. You see the whole of life is a battle, a destruction and compromise as long as we are on this material plane. So the true position seems to be, that in certain environments and stages of evolution, we have to do an amount of injury to others that we cannot avoid. So while we thus live we must eat, some of flesh and others of the vegetable kingdom. Neither class is wholly right nor wrong, it becomes wrong when we deliberately without actual need destroy the lives of animals because they are in the way of our selfish progress we must become more aware of all the creatures that live here with us.

Man, like all other material being, lives at the expense of some others, even our death is brought about by the defeat of one party of microbe(cancer, tuberculosis, aids) who are devoured by the others, who then themselves turn around and get devoured them self. This is why at the beginning I pointed out how difficult it is to follow this idea unfortunately the real problem boils down in the way man handles the world today with world hunger, ecology and the problem with the environment which is being affected by the demand of meat and its by-products, because of deforestation that is needed in order to feed animals and humans. I will get deeper into this issue in later chapters.

Religious

Hinduism, Christianity, Jainism, Buddhism, Islam, Judaism, Hare Krishna, and Sikhism

Vegetarianism and Religion are strongly linked in a number of religions that originated in the Eastern and western part of the world each with their own traditions and customs. All major Religions of the world have something to say about animals and their relationship with man, and of course whether we should make them part of our diets. In ancient India (Hinduism, Buddhism, Jainism, Hare Krishna, and Sikhism) Indian major religions (Eastern traditions) are much more critical on the subject of animal sacrifice because of their believe and opinion on the double nature of humans and animals. They believe that just as we have evolved physically, humans and animals also evolve spiritually, evolving from the mineral kingdom, to the vegetable kingdom with the same spirit or soul, and eventually to animal and then to human in a spiritual form. This they call a spiritual evolution of sentient beings, and stating that they are all living beings in their own ways, and levels of existence. This in reality makes things a lot more difficult when you look at things from a humanitarian point of view.

When it comes to the Religions of the Western traditions (Judaism, Christianity, and Islam) Aramaic Religions these Religions are not as critical as the ones that originated from ancient India their holy books give a very mixed message when it comes to animal being sacrificed for mans diet. Their God does not seem to care too much about the feelings of animals which put a big question mark on the idea that if he meant for them to be killed and eaten by man why did he create them full of feelings and emotions and individual needs. According to this view he created them for man to do whatever he wants to do with them.

Ancient Indian Religions

Hinduism

*T*he suffering of all beings according to Hinduism is believed to arise from craving and desire, conditioned by the karmic effects of both animal and human action. Hinduism holds that such influences affect he who permits the slaughter of an animal, he who kills it, he who cuts it up, he who buys it, he who sells meat, he who cooks it, he who serves it up, and he who eats it. They must all be considered the slayers of the animal. The question of religious duties towards the animals and of negative Karma incurred from violence against them is discussed in detail in Hindu scriptures and religious law books, they believe that every action that man has against animals recoils back to him in a equal manner in this life or in a another live after this one.

These texts strongly condemn the slaughter of animals and meat eating unless it happens in the context of the appropriate sacrifice ritual administered by priests. The Mahabharata allows people who are warriors by profession (Kshatriyas) to hunt and to eat meat "acquired by expenditure of prowess", but opposes such activities in the case of hermits who must strictly abstain them self from any violent toward everything in the world including the whole of the animal kingdom, and from people from regular walk of life they have to abstain from flesh eating. We can gather from what has been said that the Hindus them self's have a mixed message when it comes to animals and who can eat them and who cannot.

Jainism

Vegetarianism in Jainism is based on the principle of nonviolence like in Hinduism, but it is stricter than in the main Hindu traditions and mandatory for everyone. Jains are either lacto-vegetarians or very strict vegans they do not slaughter the cows after the cows can't produce more milk. No use or consumption of products obtained from dead animals is allowed. Moreover Jains try to avoid unnecessary injury to plants and for subtle life forms; minuscule organisms. The goal is to cause as little violence to living things as possible, hence they avoid eating roots, tubers and anything that involves uprooting (and thus eventually killing) a plant to obtain food they are the ones that come the closes to the humane principle of vegetarianism in the East.

Food which contains even small particles of the bodies of dead animals or eggs is absolutely unacceptable, Jains go out of their way so as not to hurt even small insects and other tiny animals, because they are convinced that harm caused by carelessness is as reprehensible as harm caused by deliberate action. Hence they take great pains to make sure that no minuscule animals are injured by the preparation of their meals and in the process of eating and drinking.

Traditionally Jains have been prohibited from drinking unfiltered water. In the past, when wells or baolis were used for the water source, the cloth used for filtering used to be reversed and some filtered water was poured over it to return the organisms to the original body of water. This practice termed as 'jivani' or 'bilchhavani', is no longer possible because of the use of pipes for water supply.

Jains today may also filter faucet water in the traditional fashion, and a few Jains continue to follow the filtering process even with commercial mineral or bottled drinking water.

Jains make considerable efforts not to injure plants in everyday life as far as possible. They admit that plants must be destroyed for the sake of food, but they only accept such violence inasmuch as it is indispensable for human survival, and there are special instructions for preventing unnecessary violence against plants. Jains don't eat root vegetables such as potatoes, onions, roots, carrots, and tubers, because tiny life forms are injured when the plant is pulled up and because the bulb is seen as a living being, as it is able to sprout. Also, consumption of most root vegetables involves uprooting & killing the entire plant. Whereas consumption of most terrestrial vegetables doesn't kill the plant (it lives on after plucking the vegetables or it was seasonally supposed to wither away anyway). Honey is forbidden, as its collection would amount to violence against the bees.

Food items that have started to decay are prohibited.

Traditionally cooking or eating at night was discouraged because insects are attracted to the lamps or fire at night. Strict Jains take the vow (called anastamita or anthau) of not eating after sunset.

Strict Jains do not consume food which has been fermented overnight, as it would be considered 'stale'. Hence, they may not consume yogurt or dhokla & idly batter unless they've been freshly set on the same day. During some specific fasting periods in the Jain religious, Jains refrain from consuming any green colored vegetables which have chlorophyll pigment such as okra, leafy vegetables. As can be seen there is no limit as to how far this situation can be taken and the level of sacrifice that is needed, and still animals will fall to the routine of daily living.

Buddhism

*T*he Buddha made distinction between killing an animal and consumption of meat, stressing that it is immoral conduct that makes one impure, not the food one eats. At one point the Buddha specifically refused to institute vegetarianism. There were, however, rules prohibiting certain types of meat, such as human, leopard or elephant. Monks are also prohibited from consuming meat if they witnessed the animal's death or know it was killed specifically for them.

On the other hand, the Buddha in certain Mahayana sutras strongly denounces the eating of meat. In the Mahayana Mahaparinirvana Sutra, the Buddha states that "the eating of meat extinguishes the seed of great compassion", adding that all and every kind of meat and fish consumption (even of animals already found dead) is prohibited by him. The Buddha goes on to emphasize that meat-eating cannot coexist with the great compassion and calls for not just a vegetarian, but a vegan lifestyle. The Lankavatara Sutra (a Mahayana scripture), in particular, devotes an entire chapter to the Buddha's response to the request of a disciple named Mahamati to "teach us as to the merit and vice of meat-eating." A long passage in the Lankavatara Sutra shows the Buddha weighing strongly in favor of vegetarianism, since the eating of the flesh of fellow sentient beings is said by him to be incompatible with the compassion a Bodhisattva should strive to cultivate. Several other Mahayana sutras also emphatically prohibit the consumption of meat.

In the modern Buddhist world, attitudes toward vegetarianism vary by location. In China and Vietnam, monks typically eat no meat. In Japan or Korea some schools do not eat meat, while most do. Theravadins in Sri Lanka and South-east Asia do not practice vegetarianism. All Buddhists however, including monks, are allowed to practice vegetarianism if they wish to do so. Experts have estimated that worldwide about half of all Buddhists are vegetarian.

The Buddha describes his family being wealthy enough to provide non-vegetarian meals even to his servants. After becoming the Buddha, he accepted any food offered with respect as alms, including meat, but there is no reference of him eating meat during his seven years as an ascetic.

In this particular sutta, Buddha instructs to a monk or nun to accept, without any discrimination, whatever food is offered in receiving alms offered with good will, including meat, whereas the Buddha declares the meat trade to be wrong livelihood.

In Buddhism, what is most important is to recognize that being alive, by its very nature, is the cause of direct or indirect suffering and death to other beings (samsara). One should avoid gluttony and greedy consumption, while maintaining a healthy diet and lifestyle which is conducive to attaining enlightenment. In the Pali Canon, the Buddha refused suggestion by Devadatta to institute vegetarianism in the monastic code. In most Buddhist branches, one may adopt vegetarianism if one so wishes but it is not considered skillful practice to verbally attack another person for eating meat.

In the Pali Canon, Buddha explicitly declared meat-eating to be karma neutral. Buddha's advice on meat eating was directed specifically to monks. In his comment, he stated that monks and nuns are not allowed to eat meat if they have seen, heard or suspect that the meat was killed specifically for them.

The Tibetan position is that it is not necessary to be vegetarian if one practices Vajrayana, but that it is necessary to be vegetarian if one practices the Mahayana path. The 14th Dalai Lama and other esteemed lamas invite their audiences to adopt vegetarianism when they can. When asked in recent years what he thinks of vegetarianism, the 14th Dalai Lama has said: "It is wonderful. We must absolutely promote vegetarianism." The Dalai Lama tried becoming a vegetarian and promoted vegetarianism. In 1999, it was published that the Dalai Lama would only be vegetarian every other day and partakes of meat regularly. When he is in Dharamsala, he is vegetarian, but not necessarily when he is outside Dharamsala. Paul McCartney has taken him to task for this and wrote to him to urge him to return to strict vegetarianism, but "The Dalai Lama replied, saying that his doctors had told him he needed meat, so I wrote back saying they were wrong."

So you see the idea of vegetarianism in the Buddhist religion has a very mixed message it's up to the individual to decide which path to follow.

Sikhism

F ollowers of Sikhism do not have a preference for meat or vegetarian consumption. There are two views on initiated or "Amritdhari Sikhs" and meat consumption. "Amritdhari" Sikhs (i.e. those that follow the Sikh Rehat Maryada (the Official Sikh Code of Conduct) can eat meat (provided it is not Kutha meat). "Amritdhari" that belong to some Sikh sects (e.g. Akhand Kirtani Jatha, Damdami Taksal, Namdhari, Rarionwalay, etc.) are vehemently against the consumption of meat and eggs. In the case of meat, the Sikh Gurus have indicated their preference for a simple diet, which could include meat or be vegetarian. Passages from the Guru Granth Sahib (the holy book of Sikhs, also known as the Adi Granth) say that fools argue over this issue. Guru Nanak said that over consumption of food (Lobh, Greed) involves a drain on the Earth's resources and thus on life. The tenth guru, Guru Gobind

Singh, prohibited the Sikhs from the consumption of halal or Kutha (any ritually slaughtered meat) meat because of the Sikh belief that sacrificing an animal in the name of God is mere ritualism (something to be avoided).

Hare Krishna

In the last 40 or more years the Hare Krishna movement has introduced these ethical considerations around the world. Srila Prabhupada, the movement's founder-acarya (spiritual master) had a great influence on people of all walk of live especially with very famous people. Although I did not agree with him in every aspect I can safely say that the Krishna movement had a very big influence in my decision about becoming a vegetarian. once stated, "In the Manu-samhita the concept of a life for a life is sanctioned, and it is actually observed throughout the world. Similarly, there are other laws which state that one cannot even kill an ant without being responsible. Since we cannot create, we have no right to kill any living entity, and therefore man-made laws that distinguish between killing a man and killing an animal are imperfect . . . According to the laws of God, killing an animal is as punishable as killing a man. Those who draw distinctions between the two are concocting their own laws. Even in the Ten Commandments it is prescribed, 'Thou shall not kill.' This is a perfect law, but by discriminating and speculating men distort it. 'I shall not kill man, but I shall kill animals.' In this way people cheat themselves and inflict suffering on themselves and others."

Emphasizing the Vedic conception of the unity of all life, Srila Prabhupada then stated, "Everyone is God's creature, although in different bodies or dresses. God is considered the one supreme father. A father may have many children, and some may be intelligent and others not very intelligent, but if an intelligent son tells his father, 'My brother is not very intelligent; let me kill him,' will the father agree? . . . Similarly, if God is the supreme father, why should He sanction the killing of animals who are also His sons?"

Abrahamic Religions

Judaism, Christianity, Islam

*A*brahamic religions are religions which share the patriarch Abraham in their religious lineage, although he plays different roles in different Abrahamic religions. Islam, Christianity, and Judaism are all considered to be Abrahamic religions, as Abraham appears in the religious texts of all of these faiths, also the Druze, Bahai, Samaritans, and others are sometimes considered to be Abrahamic religions as well. All told, over half of the people in the world identify themselves as members of an Abrahamic religion, and they are the religions of the Western traditions.

In addition to sharing the figure of Abraham, numerous other figures can be found in the tradition of all of the Abrahamic religions, such as Noah, and these religions share several common traits, as well. All Abrahamic religions are monotheist, believing in one god. In the case of Judaism and Islam, Abraham is viewed as a literal father of the religion, in the direct lineage of various prophets and other important religious figures, and in the case of Christianity, Abraham plays the role of a spiritual father, because Christianity is derived from Judaism.

Judaism

*H*ow does Judaism view vegetarianism? Is it favored or discouraged by the Torah?

While Jewish Dietary Laws originated in the Bible (Leviticus 11 and Deuteronomy 17), they have been codified and interpreted over the centuries by rabbinical authorities.

Upon his creation, Adam, the first man, was told by God: "Behold, I have given you every seed-bearing herb which is upon the surface of the entire earth and every tree that has seed-bearing fruit; it will be yours for food. This was the first instruction given to Jews from their God about what his diet should be and basically what his relationship was going to be between them and the animal kingdom.

Several thousand (over 1600) years later, upon surviving the devastation of the great Flood, caused by their God when he repented to have created man admitting his mistake for creating them. When Noah and his family the only survivors of the flood leaves the Ark, and is told by his God, "Every moving thing that lives shall be yours to eat; like the green vegetation, I have given you everything. So there was a big change in the order from God to his people(Jews) about what exactly he wanted them to do when it came to their diet, and their responsibility when it comes to their relationship with the rest of his creation.

It would seem that God's original (and ideal) plan was that we should not eat meat. One problem with this approach is that many statements in the Torah imply that meat eating is ideal and encouraged, for example to honor the Shabbat and the holidays.

So what is the deal? Would God rather we be vegetarians like Adam or meat eaters like Noah, the problem with this is that the Jewish God is a God of change, the Torah is a book full of changes that come directly from God himself.

The 15th century philosopher Rabbi Yosef Albo, author of Sefer HaIkarim ("The Book of Principles"), understands God's instructions to Adam as an implication that the original Godly plan was that man should refrain from killing and eating meat. In his view, the killing of animals is a cruel and furious act, ingraining these negative traits in the human character; in addition, the meat of certain animals coarsens the heart and deadens its spiritual sensitivity.

The people of the first generations mistook this, however, to mean that humans and animals were equal, with equal expectations and standards. This led to the degeneration of society into violence and corruption; for if the human being is but another beast, then killing a man is the equivalent of killing of an animal. It was this attitude and behavior which prompted God to cleanse the world with the Great Flood. But the problem with **this** is that Gods new order brought about more violence to the world for now he told the Jewish people that it's ok for them to kill sentient beings like themselves for their own selfish use. From this it is gathered that Judaism is definitely not a vegetarian religion for it is written in its holy book the Torah, and any Jew that wants to be a vegetarian is doing it against it, for this was a direct order from his God.

Christianity

We know that any religion that basis their believe in the holy Bible or the Torah are bound to the law and command that was given to them by their God, but we all know that the Bible has a totally mixed message when it comes to this topic. So the problem is not what the bible says but what each individual feels personally about what to accept, because in reality we all know that the real message is against vegetarianism. There are lots of people today that want to have their cake and eat it at the same time, wanting to be Christian and vegetarians at the same time justifying them self through the bible.

According to some interpretations of the Bible, raw veganism was the original diet of humankind in the form given to Adam and Eve by God in Genesis 1:29, "And God said, Behold, I have given you every herb bearing seed, which is upon the face of all the earth, and every tree, in the which is the fruit of a tree yielding seed; to you it shall be for **meat**."

Many Christian Vegetarians believe that upon the return of Christ, the world will return to vegetarianism. Even thought the bible is full of statements where Jesus himself ate animal and feed them to others.

While vegetarianism is not a common practice in current western Christian thought and culture, the concept and practice has substantial scriptural and historical support. According to the Bible, in the beginning, humans and animals were vegetarian (Genesis 1:29–30). Immediately after the Flood, God permitted the eating of meat, however, some maintain that God permitted the consumption of meat only temporarily because all plants had been destroyed as a result of the flood, despite the lack of any reference to this in Genesis itself. We must also remember that Noah only had a pair of every living animal on board the ark and if they started to kill and eat them right away how could they multiply on the face of the earth.

Furthermore, centuries after Noah God did not change his idea about the consumption of meat he only specified which ones to eat and the ones to avoid. Leviticus 11 also records God giving the Israelites rules about what types of meat may be eaten, logically requiring that certain meats were acceptable. So it's pretty clear what Gods intentions were after the flood when it came to the diet he wanted for his Jewish people to adapt.

The Old Testament also says that God commanded the Israelites to eat meat on some occasions. During the Exodus out of Egypt and the first Passover, God commanded all of the Israelites to slaughter a Passover lamb and eat it giving the clear message that it's ok to kill for some cause, whether for dietary reason or for some sacrifice in his name. This was to be a lasting tradition (Exodus 12:24).

Some Christians believe that the Bible explains that, in the future, humans and animals will return to vegetarianism. Some people believe that the Book of Daniel also specifically promotes vegetarianism as beneficial. Daniel specifically refuses the king's "meat" Daniel 1:8–16 However, current common theology argues that in this instance Daniel is rejecting food that is considered to be unholy by his faith or not kosher or (eating food that had been sacrificed to pagan gods), and not meat per se.

All four Gospels offer that Jesus gave fish to others (Matthew 14:17-21, Mark 6:38-44, Luke 24:42-43, John 6:9-12), and according to Luke 24:41-43 Jesus ate fish himself after his resurrection; in addition, Luke's Acts of the Apostles portrays a story where the Apostle Peter has a vision where God declares previously unclean meat as "clean" Acts 10:7-16 and orders Peter to "kill and eat",this can be also a mixed message referring to the accepting of the gentiles into the order of Jews. Nevertheless, a number of Christian leaders, both ancient and modern, observe that vegetarianism was and is a sincere part of Christian faith.

Vegetarianism appears to have been a point of contention within early Christian circles. Within the Bible's New Testament, the Apostle Paul appears to ridicule vegetarians, arguing that people of weak faith eat only vegetables Romans 14:1–4 (although he also warns believers to stop passing judgment on one another when it comes to food in verse

13). Within Luke's Acts of the Apostles, Luke recounts that the Jerusalem Council authorized that (at least for Gentile Christians) it was acceptable to eat meat Acts 15:19–20.

In some Christian communities partial fasting, for example during Lent, resembles vegetarianism since meat and dairy products are forbidden for a temporary period. For some groups, such as Catholics, seafood is permitted during these periods of fasting. A basic difference to other forms of vegetarianism is that Lent has spiritual connotation, not environmental or animal welfare reasons. Also, abstaining from meat and dairy products during Lent is intended to be temporary, lasting only until the season is over, not a permanent way of life.

The Seventh-day Adventists present a health message that recommends vegetarianism and expects abstinence from pork, shellfish and other foods proscribed as "unclean" in Leviticus. Another denomination with common origin, the Seventh Day Adventist Reform Movement requires vegetarianism as a test of fellowship, with many of its members being practicing vegans as well even though their idea is mostly based on a dietary and healthy issue.

Muslims (Islam)

According to scholars the Prophet Mohammed, although not a vegetarian, did prefer to eat vegetarian foods and had a great love and compassion for animals. His favorite foods consisted of yogurt with butter or nuts, cucumbers with dates, pomegranates, grapes and figs. He was known to have quoted: "Where there is an abundance of vegetables, a host of angels will descend on that place."

The Prophet recognized that each person is a unique autonomous individual with his or her own personality. When giving advice to individual Companions, he would specifically tailor the advice according to that person's own characteristics. He did not enforce any overbearing uniformity on the people. Especially when it came to eating, he recognized that different people have different tastes. And for that matter, not even the Prophet and his Companions ate meat all the time; it was only once in a while that they did, not every day.

Like most of the world's religions (except Jainism), modern Islam does not fully support vegetarianism, although certain Muslim sects such as the Shiites and Sufis have vegetarian followers. Throughout the African, Middle Eastern and Southeast Asian parts of the Islamic World, meat is a rarity, making vegetarianism a necessity and not a choice.

The Qur'an however permits a Muslim to have non-vegetarian food. The following Qur'an verses are proof of this fact:

"O ye who believe! Fulfill (all) obligations. Lawful unto you (for food) are all four-footed animals with the exceptions named." [Al-Qur'an 5:1]

"And cattle He has created for you (men): from them Ye derive warmth, and numerous benefits, And of their (meat) ye eat."

[Al-Qur'an 16:5]

"And in cattle (too) ye have an instructive example: From within their bodies we produce (milk) for you to drink; there are, in them, (besides), numerous (other) benefits for you; and of their (meat) ye eat."

[Al-Qur'an 23:21]

The one overall guideline on food that the Prophet gave was: Eat of what is halâl and what is agreeable to you. That says it all. Within the wide range of halâl food, each individual can choose to eat whatever suits him or her. Although technically "halâl" means simply "permitted," the opposite of "haram," we most often hear it used in reference to food. Often described as Muslim kosher, halâl and kosher rules and prohibitions do differ despite some similarities.

If people want to follow the Prophet's Sunnah of eating, consider this: The Prophet ate what he liked and he left aside what he didn't like. That's all we vegetarians are doing! Furthermore, he never coerced anyone else into eating what they didn't like. How about imitating this Sunnah? There was a Bedouin tribe whose custom it was to eat lizards, and the Prophet never forbade them from doing so. But he himself would never eat a lizard. This shows that just because something is "halâl," that doesn't require you to eat it if you don't want to.

The bottom line is: no one has the authority to dictate to you what halâl food you can choose to put into your body. Islamic law is completely neutral on this issue; it is only a private matter for each individual to decide for his or her self whatever you consider to be morally wrong to you from that you should reframe, but you should not criticize anybody for feeling different.

As we can see that even all major Religions are divided among themselves when it comes to vegetarianism, we can appreciate that at some time or another they all have something to say about animals being sacrifices for the use of mans need.

Vitamin B12(colamabin)

*I*t's incredible how mush learning I have done since I took up the task of writing about vegetarianism once again. For it not only involves vegetarianism but the whole of mans health, diet, and ethics when it comes to his place in the world today. Throughout all this research I have found that one of the most important things is for us to have a full understanding of our place in this beautiful planet that we all live in and to try and understand our duty in its complexity.

Throughout all this research I learned about the most complex vitamin that involves the human body (vitamin B12). That is why I took a whole lengthy chapter in what I think is the most important vitamin not only for vegans but also for non-vegetarians. I believe that the complete understanding of this vitamin will clear up all of the questions concerning mans real physiological dietary needs, and where he falls in nature and the animal kingdom. It helps to understand whether he is an herbivore, omnivore, or carnivorous animal by nature by exploring his dietary needs and from where is he supposed to get all his nutrients and vitamins. Please pay close attention to this chapter for I can't stress enough the importance of this very important vitamin.

Even thought vegetarianism is present in all geographic areas of the world and it's been around for thousands of years, only in the past 60 or so years (1948) was this very important vitamin recognized and the important role it plays when it comes to the human body. So it's only been a few years that it was recognized that vegetarians have had consistently lower vitamin B-12 concentrations than do non—vegetarians and those vegetarians are at greater risk of vitamin B-12 deficiency than are non-vegetarians.

I would like to make a comment here and say that all those famous people from 1948 and back that made statements about how healthy is a vegan diet did not know or even have a clue about this most important vitamin and how deficient and harmful was this diet that they were promoting without the supplements we know about today. Because vitamin B-12 is produced in nature only by vitamin B-12–producing microorganisms, vegans must receive vitamin B-12 solely from dietary supplements. Although there are abundant vitamin B-12 producing bacteria that colonize the large bowel in man, that organ is too distal to allow normal vitamin B-12 absorption. Herbivores obtain vitamin B-12 primarily from plants contaminated with nitrogen-fixing, vitamin B-12 producing bacteria that grow in roots and nodes of legumes and from plants contaminated with feces. The ruminant animals get most of theirs from bacteria in their rumen through the special ability of eating their food than returning it back and being broken down by microorganism and returned back as cud with enough vitamin B12 and other nutrients. Carnivorous lower animals receive their vitamin B-12 by eating insects and other animals and via coprophagy (the ability to eat their own feces) we will understand all this as the chapter develops.

Definition

Vitamin B12, vitamin B12 or vitamin B-12,

Also called cobalamin, it is a water soluble vitamin and a member of the B complex with a key role in the normal functioning of the brain and nervous system, and for the formation of blood. It is normally involved in the metabolism of every cell of the body, especially affecting DNA synthesis and regulation, but also fatty acid synthesis and energy production. As the largest and most structurally complicated vitamin it is exclusively synthesized by bacteria and is found primarily in meat, eggs, and dairy products, it can be produced industrially only through bacterial fermentation-synthesis. There has been considerable research done in the proposed plant source of vitamin B12, fermented soya products, seaweeds tempeh, miso, shoyu, tamari, and algae such as spirulina have all been suggested as containing significant B12. However, the present consensus is that any B12 present in plant foods is likely to be unavailable to humans and so these foods should not be relied upon as safe sources of the vitamin. I will get into a more detailed explanation why there has been a misunderstanding about B12 found in plants.

Vitamin B12 consists of a class of chemically-related compounds (vitamers), all of which have vitamin activity. It contains the biochemically rare element cobalt. Biosynthesis of the basic structure of the vitamin in nature is only accomplished by simple organisms such as some bacteria and algae.

Deficiency and Function

Methylcobalamin is the preferred type of vitamin B-12. Cyanocobalamin must be converted to methyl or Adenosyl cobalamin by the body, and it's needed for fat and carbohydrate metabolism and formation of blood cells. Deficiency results in mental confusion, anemia, homocystenia,

Brain damage, tinnitus, asthma, and depression. B-12 deficiency leads to heart risk and may benefit multiple sclerosis patients. Deficiency is widespread in people over sixty years of age. Alcohol, estrogen, oral contraceptives, sleeping pills interfere with utilization of the bodies use of the vitamin. Natural sources are liver, beef, pork, eggs, milk, and milk by-products, except where soil is deficient in cobalt. The vitamin needs calcium for the body's absorption. Microwave cooking destroys B-12 of the food that is cooked or heated in these machines.

In a study of 64 patients taking 500 mcg of oral B-12 daily the lowest absorption rate was 1.8 mcg. Since this is less than the 2 mcg daily requirement a 500 mcg dosage would be insufficient.

In most cases the mean absorption rate is 1.2 percent of intake. B-12 is widely available in 1000 and 2000 microgram potencies. No known toxicity as of now has been reported.

Vitamin B12's primary functions are in the formation of red blood cells and the maintenance of a healthy nervous system. B12 is necessary for the rapid synthesis of DNA during cell division. This is especially important in tissues where cells are dividing rapidly, particularly the bone marrow tissues responsible for red blood cell formation. If B12 deficiency occurs, DNA production is disrupted and abnormal cells called mega oblasts occur. This results in anemia. Symptoms include excessive tiredness, breathlessness, listlessness, pallor, and poor resistance to infection. Older people with vitamin B12 deficiency benefit from taking vitamin B12 supplements because the deficiency usually results from difficulty absorbing the vitamin from meat. They can absorb the vitamin more easily from supplements than from meat.

Vitamin B12 can be stored in small amounts by the body. Total body store is 2-5mg in adults. Around 80% of this is stored in the liver. This is the reason why many people who become vegans can go on for a long time without the need of this vitamin and think that they can go on without it and think they are healthy they should get checked.

B12 is also important in maintaining the nervous system. Nerves are surrounded by an insulating fatty sheath comprised of a complex protein called myelin. B12 plays a vital role in the metabolism of fatty acids essential for the maintenance of myelin. Prolonged B12 deficiency can lead to nerve degeneration and irreversible neurological damage.

Ultimately, neither plants nor animals are independently capable of constructing Vitamin B12.Only bacteria have the enzymes required for its synthesis. Thus, herbivorous animals must either obtain B12 from bacteria in their rumens, or (if fermenting plant material in the hindgut) by reinjection of cecotrope feces.

Vitamin B12 is found in foods that come from animals, including fish and shellfish, meat (especially liver), poultry, eggs, milk, and milk by-products.

Eggs are often mentioned as a good B12 source, but they also contain a factor (avidin) that blocks absorption of the vitamin from the body. Certain insects such as termites contain B12 produced by their gut bacteria, in a way analogous to ruminant animals.

While lacto-ovo vegetarians usually get enough B12 through consuming dairy products, vegans will lack B12 unless they consume multivitamin supplements or B12-fortified foods. Examples of fortified foods include fortified breakfast cereals, fortified soy products, fortified energy bars, and fortified nutritional yeast, fortified means that it is added to the food not that it is a part of it, this is something that has to be clear for many people think B12 is natural in these food and don't read the labels to verify if it was added. According to the UK Vegan Society, the present consensus is that any B12 present in plant foods is likely to be unavailable to humans because B12 analogues can compete with B12 and inhibit metabolism.

Several food sources of vitamin B12 are listed in Table 1.

Table 1: Selected Food Sources of Vitamin B12

Food	Micrograms (mcg) per serving	Percent DV*
Liver, beef, braised, 1 slice	48.0	800
Clams, cooked, breaded and fried, 3 ounces	34.2	570
Breakfast cereals, fortified with 100% of the DV for vitamin B12, 1 serving	6.0	100
Trout, rainbow, wild, cooked, 3 ounces	5.4	90
Salmon, sockeye, cooked, 3 ounces	4.9	80
Trout, rainbow, farmed, cooked, 3 ounces	4.2	50
Beef, top sirloin, broiled, 3 ounces	2.4	40
Cheeseburger, double patty and bun,	1.9	30
Breakfast cereals, fortified with 25% of the DV for vitamin B12, 1 serving	1.5	25
Yogurt, plain, 1 cup	1.4	25
Haddock, cooked, 3 ounces	1.2	20
Tuna, white, 3 ounces	1.0	15
Milk, 1 cup	0.9	15
Cheese, Swiss, 1 ounce	0.9	15
Beef taco, 1 taco	0.8	13
Ham, cured, roasted, 3 ounces	0.6	10
Egg, large, 1 whole	0.6	10
Chicken, roasted, ½ breast	0.3	6

Recommended Intakes

*I*ntake recommendations for vitamin B12 and other nutrients are provided in the Dietary Reference Intakes (DRIs) developed by the Food and Nutrition Board (FNB) at the Institute of Medicine (IOM) of the National Academies (formerly National Academy of Sciences). These values, which vary by age and gender, include:

Recommended Dietary Allowance (RDA): average daily level of intake sufficient to meet the nutrient requirements of nearly all (97%–98%) healthy individuals.

Adequate Intake (AI): established when evidence is insufficient to develop an RDA and is set at a level assumed to ensure nutritional adequacy.

Tolerable Upper Intake Level (UL): maximum daily intake unlikely to cause adverse health effects

Table 1 lists the current RDAs for vitamin B12 in micrograms (mcg) for infants aged 0 to 12 months, the FNB established an AI for vitamin B12 that is equivalent to the mean intake of vitamin B12 in healthy, breastfed infants.

Table 1: Recommended Dietary Allowances (RDAs) for Vitamin B12

Age	Male	Female	Pregnancy	Lactation
Birth to 6 months*	0.4 mcg	same		
7-12 months*	0.5 mcg	same		
1-3 years	0.9 mcg	same		
4-8 years	1.2 mcg	same		
9-13 years	1.8 mcg	same		
14+ years	2.4 mcg	2.4 mcg	2.6 mcg	2.8 mcg

Dietary supplements

*I*n dietary supplements, vitamin B12 is usually present as cyanocobalamin, a form that the body readily converts to the active forms methylcobalamin and 5-deoxyadenosylcobalamin. Dietary supplements can also contain methylcobalamin and other forms of vitamin B12, always check your labels to see that one of these is present.

Existing evidence does not suggest any differences among forms with respect to absorption or bioavailability. However the body's ability to absorb vitamin B12 from dietary supplements is largely limited by the capacity of intrinsic factor. For example, only about 10 mcg of a 500 mcg oral supplement is actually absorbed in healthy people.

In addition to oral dietary supplements, vitamin B12 is available in sublingual preparations as tablets or lozenges. These preparations are frequently marketed as having superior bioavailability, although evidence suggests no difference in efficacy between oral and sublingual forms.

Bacteria in the Large Intestine

A re Intestinal Bacteria a Reliable Source of B12 for humans?

It has long been assumed that B12 is produced by bacteria in the large intestine of animals, the colon, but since B12 is produced below the ileum, where B12 is absorbed, in the colon it is not available for absorption and the vitamin does not have the ability to travel up here it could be available for absorption. Because there is no absorption in this part of the body only in ruminant animals is it available. This theory is reinforced by the fact that many species of totally or primarily vegetarian animals eat their feces, and plants infected with feces. It is surmised that eating feces allows them to obtain B12 on their diets of plant foods.

Bacteria present in the large intestine are able to synthesize B12 in most animals primarily mammals. In the past, it has been thought that the B12 produced by these colonic bacteria could be absorbed and utilized by humans. However, the bacteria that produces B12 are too far down the intestine for absorption to occur, B12 not being absorbed through the colon lining.

Human feces can contain significant B12. A study has shown that a group of Iranian vegans obtained adequate B12 from unwashed vegetables which had been fertilized with human manure a practice that is well known in European countries. Fecal contamination of vegetables and other plant foods can make a significant contribution to dietary needs, particularly in areas where hygiene standards may be different, and they fertilize their vegetables with animal and human feces pulled out from dry latrines, and by not washing their vegetables they absorbed the B12 on the surface of the vegetables. Sometimes confusing people thinking that the plants are the ones that produce the vitamins. This may be responsible for the lack of anemia due to B12 deficiency in vegan communities where these hygienic principals are applied.

In many species, such as the rabbit, stool eating (coprophagy) is a normal behavior that provides a variety of vital nutrients, including B-complex vitamins. In the case of rats, 5% to 50% of their fecal output is eaten, providing them with an important source of thiamine and vitamin K. Although dogs do not need to eat feces for good health, when they are fed a thiamine-deficient diet, dogs will engage in coprophagy to stave off physical symptoms and attenuate neurological signs of thiamine deficiency, at least temporarily. In horses, foals less than 20 weeks of age show a preference for their mother's feces, which they eat. Equine coprophagy may provide foals with various nutrients (vitamins and proteins) and beneficial bacterial flora needed for digestion. Mother dogs instinctively elicit elimination and ingest their puppies' excrements from birth to approximately 3 weeks of age. Adult males will also ingest feces produced by young puppies. Although dogs of all ages may show this behavior, coprophagy is particularly common among puppies and young dogs between 4 and 9 months of age. Besides eating their own feces, some dogs ingest feces of other dogs and animals, especially cat and horse droppings. Most dogs actively explore the droppings of other dogs and animals, but, for some dogs, something in the feces is sufficiently attractive for them to go further and eat it. There has always been a big confusion when it comes to whether animals especially humans are vegetarians. There have been lots of things written about this subject trying to prove that man physiologically is a vegetarian animal by nature and that the eating of any kind of animal is a totally unnatural habit. There still remains the problem of this most important vitamin B12 and how important it is to the human body. The main question is from what natural source in nature did our ancestors acquired this most important vitamin if they were complete vegetarians. According to science today it is only produced by bacteria and not from anything in the vegetable kingdom so how did humans and other animals acquire it in nature if they were to be herbivore. Scientists and anthropologies today have found that many animals that were thought to be vegetarians are not complete vegetarians for example chimpanzees, pandas, and all primates have been seen killing other animals and insects for food and favoring really ripe fruits in order to eat the insects that are found in them and then eating them in order to find a good source of vitamins and nutrients that are not found in any vegetable.

I believe that man is an omnivore with a diet of about 70% or more based on fruits and vegetable making him more of a vegetarian then a carnivore as stated above making him an omnivore by nature. If we compare man physiologically to all animals we can appreciate that he is more of a vegetarian animal than a carnivore but not totally vegetarian for as stated above he also has many features and physical needs of a carnivores.